E-Discovery Nuts and Bolts:

101 Tips for the Healthcare Professional

Dale Newton, M.D.,

Anthony Johnson, LL.M

FORWARD

Effective January 1, 2014, federal mandates for healthcare and digital record-keeping was required for public and private healthcare providers. A key provision of the American Recovery and Reinvestment Act of 2009 went into effect and healthcare providers across the country are failing to comply.

The American Recovery and Reinvestment Act also includes financial incentives for healthcare provides who provide meaningful use of electronic health records (EHR). HER is not only a more comprehensive patient history than EMR, the latter of which contains a patient's medical history from just one practice, but also the end-goal of the federal mandate. "Meaningful use" of HER, as defined by HealthIT.gov, consists of using digital medical and health records to achieve the following:

- Improve quality, safety, efficiency, and reduce health disparities
- Engage patients and family
- Improve care coordination, and population and public health

- Maintain privacy and security of patient health information

Penalties also exist for non-compliance. EP's who haven't implemented EMR/HER systems and demonstrated their meaningful use by 2015 will experience a 1% reduction in Medicare reimbursements, and rates of reduction will likely rise annually thereafter.

Not surprisingly, the EMR/EMH mandate is already effecting significant growth in E-Discovery, or "Electronic Data Discovery", an interdisciplinary field of study that merges information technology, healthcare, and the legalities thereof.

Today, there is a vast "disconnect" between the legal profession, healthcare, and technology. Most legal professionals today have a total lack of understanding of "technology" concepts as they relate to discovery of electronic information. For physicians who either have not adopted a certified HER/EMR systems or cannot demonstrate "meaningful use" bye the EMR deadline in 2015, Medicare reimbursements will be reduced by 1%. The deduction rate increases in subsequent years by 2%

in 2016, 3% in 2017, 4% in 2018, and up to 95% depending on future adjustments.

According to EMRandHipaa.com, an average AAFP (American Academy of Family Physicians) user is reimbursed 20% by Medicare. This means that overall, a private practice with $500,000 of annual income that fails to meet the electronic medical records mandate will lose $1,000 in payments in 2015, $2,000 in 2016, and so on.

Meeting the government's mandate and electronic medical records deadline will not be easy for everyone in the health industry. "Rural hospitals and small, independent physician practices will have a harder time meeting the digital medical records requirements. But the incentives and potential penalties under the Recovery Act have made it clear that they no longer can put off the challenging task of parting with their paper charts," writes the Milwaukee Journal Sentinel.

On the other hand, as part of the American Recovery and Reinvestment Act, physicians can receive up to $44,000 in Medicare incentive payments beginning in 2011 for implementing EMR and systems. The EMR systems will help to provide physicians with a "litigation readiness" program to protect themselves in the event litigation becomes apparent.

There are several legal issues surrounding electronic medical records that healthcare professionals should become aware of, to wit:

- Risk for medical malpractice claims
- Likelihood of medical errors
- Vulnerability to fraud claims
- Breaches, theft and unauthorized access to protected health information
- Practical tips for healthcare leaders

We will address these concerns and other ways to reduce legal risks in the electronic medical records era by utilizing E-Discovery Project Management to ensure that your organization will have a litigation readiness program in place.

Today, all litigants have a duty to request and disclose responsive electronic evidence in their cases. Whether your cases are small or large, or whether you are solo practitioner, or part of large medical organization, discovery issues relating to ESMI ("Electronically Stored Medical Information") will have to be addressed and resolved.

The purpose of the E-Discovery Nuts and Bolts for Healthcare Professionals is to offer an overview and electronic workbook for the myriad of legal and technology issues that need to be addressed whether you are requesting or producing "electronically stored medical information" or ESMI. This workbook will provide a plan and pretrial steps in discovering and disclosing ESMI. Depending on the unique pretrial issues of your case, this plan may necessitate a different approach and should be considered on a case-by-case basis.

TABLE OF CONTENTS

101 Tips for Healthcare Professionals

CHAPTER 1

WHAT IMPACT WILL E-DISCOVERY HAVE ON THE HEALTHCARE INDUSTRY?

Electronic discovery in healthcare litigation is no longer coming to a court near you...it's already here. Rigorous e-discovery standards are already in place in the Federal Courts. On December 1, 2006, changes relating to electronically stored information (ESI) in the Federal Rules of Civil Procedure took effect. The changes to Rules 16, 26, 33, 34, 37, 45 and Form 35 provide mandates to the preservation, discoverability, production, accessibility, and costs associated with ESI which includes e-mail, word processing documents, spreadsheets, voice mail, databases, and more.

Today, all litigants have a duty to request and disclose responsive electronic evidence in their cases. Whether your cases are small or large, or whether you are a sole practitioner or a member of a large firm or healthcare organization, discovery issues relating to ESMI will have to be addressed and resolved.

Electronic discovery (e-discovery) is an area where there are numerous examples and implementations of artificial intelligence both replacing work product from lawyers and at the same time improving the experience of law practice. Much has been written, discussed, and litigated around the technology and benefit of e-discovery. The focus of most providers is to provide intelligent algorithms to find information based on concepts and key words agreed upon by the parties to the litigation. The "hot new thing" in e-discovery is the use of a higher-level artificial intelligence concept called "predictive coding".

Predictive coding is a process whereby a machine learns from watching human behavior and then applies what is learns. In addition to technical aptitude, successful predictive coding e-discovery requires skills in statistics, accounting, project management, and linguistics.

Electronic Discovery in Healthcare Litigation

A key provision of the American Recovery and Reinvestment Act of 2009 went into effect on January 1, 2014, and all public and private healthcare providers and other eligible professionals must have adopted and demonstrated "meaningful use" of electronic medical records (EMR) in order to maintain their existing Medicaid and Medicare reimbursement levels.

The American Recovery and Reinvestment Act also includes financial incentives for healthcare providers who prove meaningful use of electronic health records (EHR). EHR is not only a more comprehensive patient history than EMR, the latter of which contains a patient's medical history from just one practice, but also the end-goal of using digital medical and health records to achieve the following:

- Improve quality, safety, efficiency, and reduce health disparities
- Engage patients and family
- Improve care coordination, and population and public health
- Maintain privacy and security of patient health information

Best practices require that healthcare institutions be proactive in meeting the challenges of e-discovery. Unlike many prior defendants on the losing side of an e-discovery spoliation motion, healthcare providers are already obligated to preserve relevant information on patients for many years. The difficulty in a large institutional setting is knowing what information exists, where it is, what format it is in, and how best to preserve and produce it. Mapping all the data systems and identifying key players who control those systems will ensure a timely and cost effective means to implement a litigation hold to prevent data loss.

Preservation is the key to avoiding the harsh penalties from an e-discovery catastrophe. If the data is preserved, it can always be searched for and retrieved later. Once destroyed, it is very costly to try to recreate it from backup tapes or other secondary sources.

Healthcare providers must avoid an ad hoc method to addressing e-discovery requests. Efficient processes must be developed now to handle the growing number of e-discovery demands. Electronic discovery is rapidly expanding in medical malpractice litigation. Healthcare providers must be ready to respond. A proactive, practical approach before the e-discovery demand is received will reduce costs and the risk of a case-losing sanction.

How Technology is Changing the Practice of HealthcareLaw

Moore's Law

In 1965 Gordon E. Moore, one of the Intel founders, wrote a paper observing that the number of transistors on integrated circuits doubles approximately every two years. As it turned out, Moore's Law became a self-fulfilling prophecy—partly because the observation was based on empirical data at the time, but more importantly because the law is now used in the semiconductor industry to guide long-term planning and to set targets for research and development.

While the technology around the legal world advances at an exponential rate, the technology within the legal world, especially as it relates to lawyering (i.e., providing legal services as opposed to running a law business), is much slower.

For each new technological advance, a high level of analysis and review is needed before lawyers can implement it. Assuming Moore's Law represents the rate of technological advance for legal service consumers (i.e., doubling every two years), and assuming a slower rate of growth for legal service providers (perhaps increasing by one-half every two years), then, every two years the tension grows exponentially at a rate of 1.5 times. As that tension continues to grow, the legal services industry will find itself competing with outside providers attempting to fill the gap. This phenomenon is already taking place and, folks in the healthcare industry should not ignore it in light of the January 1, 2014 federal mandates for healthcare requiring digital record-keeping in the public and private sectors.

This e-book is designed to give you, the healthcare professional, a "nuts and bolts" guide to understanding electronic discovery and provide a roadmap to an efficient healthcare litigation readiness program. The 101 tips included herein is intended to be a quick reference guide for the healthcare professional and practitioner. Download this e-book to your phone, Kindle, iPad, iPhone or laptop computer for easy reference.

Check out these 101 tips and see for yourself how they will be your "go-to" guide for all matters in relation to electronic medical records, healthcare litigation, and litigation readiness.

CHAPTER 2

The Basics of Electronic Discovery

EDRM

Electronic Discovery Reference Model

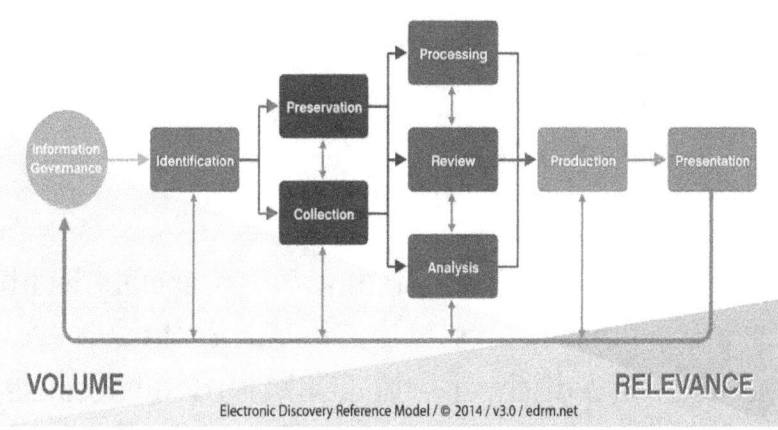

Electronic Discovery Reference Model / © 2014 / v3.0 / edrm.net

The Electronic Discovery Reference Model (EDRM) was initially conceived by George Socha, Jr., founder of Socha Consulting, LLC in St. Paul, MN, and Tom Gelbmann, managing director of Gelbmann & Associates, in Roseville, MN. The reference model divides the e-discovery process into six areas:

- Information Management
- Identification
- Preservation|Collection
- Processing|Review|Analysis
- Production
- Presentation

The EDRM identifies the functions associated with each area. It has been said that if you don't have experience in e-discovery, the EDRM is useful because it is good for showing what the issues are. The EDRM is also useful as a guide to move you along the process of identifying data and subsequently preserving that data, collecting it, processing it, and so on.

Let's take a moment to familiarize ourselves with a summary of explanations of each EDRM stage.

- Information Management: This is where a company should begin to get their electronic house in order to mitigate risk and expenses should e-discovery become an issue, from initial creation of electronically stored information through its final disposition.
- Identification: This is where you would locate potential sources of ESMI and determine its scope, breadth, and depth.
- Preservation: During this stage, you would want to ensure that ESMI is protected against inappropriate alteration or destruction.
- Collection: Collection is the gathering of ESMI for further use in the discovery process, i.e., processing, review, etc.
- Processing: This is where you would reduce the volume of ESMI and convert it, if necessary, to forms more suitable for review and analysis.
- Review: To evaluate ESMI for relevance and privilege.
- Analysis: This is where you would evaluate ESMI for content & context, including key patterns, topics, people and discussion.
- Production: To deliver ESMI to others in appropriate forms and using appropriate delivery mechanisms.

- Presentation: Displaying ESMI before audiences (at depositions, hearings, trials, etc.), especially in native and near-native forms, to elicit further information, validate existing facts or positions, or persuade an audience.

Now that we have that covered, let's take a look at the basics of E-Discovery and tie it all in...

The legal industry is slow to embrace change and adopt new practices. However, the past two decades have witnessed the dawn of the digital age and, with it, advancements in technology that have shaped the legal and healthcare landscapes. This evolving technology and recent amendments to the Federal Rules of Civil Procedure, Affordable Care Act of 2009, and The American Recovery and Reinvestment Act of 2009 have spawned a new and lucrative law practice specialty: electronic discovery. The e-discovery niche, which combines the legal expertise of attorneys with the technical skills of IT professionals, is one of the fastest growing specialties in the legal industry.

Electronic discovery has been described as the "disclosure or discovery of electronically stored information (ESMI), including the form or forms in which it should be produced..." See, <u>Junk v. Aon Corp.</u>, No. 07-4640, 2007 U.S. Dist. LEXIS 89741, at *2 n.2 (D.N.Y. Nov. 30, 2007). ESMI includes e-mail, spreadsheets, word processing documents, audio, video, instant or text messaging, personal information systems, and databases. Electronic discovery is considered to be the request, collection, review, production, and management of electronic information.

Metadata

Unlike traditional paper discovery, electronic data files will include "metadata," or what is known as additional hidden data. Metadata is defined as data providing more information about one or more aspects of the existing data. Metadata may include:

- Means of creation of the data
- Purpose of the data
- Time and date of creation
- Creation or author of data
- Location on a computer network where the data was created
- Standards used to create the data

This valuable information does not appear on the printed copy of an electronic file. Metadata is found in e-mail messages, word processing documents, spreadsheets, audio, video, and other digital files. E-mail metadata may contain who was blind copied on a message. A computer will contain information about Internet usage such as which websites were visited, when, and by whom. Metadata is an important aspect of ESMI because it may very well be more valuable than the traditional forms of evidence in building or defending a case.

Think about metadata in this concept: If you believe that your determination was based upon discrimination, you have a duty to request, and your employer would have a duty to disclose, any information relating to your job performance, performance reviews, raises, records of attendance, absenteeism, etc. Most of these documents would be kept in electronic format. The metadata would be that hidden data that would illuminate the time and date of the entry of the data, who had entered the data, what entity had entered the data, the location on the database network where the data was created, etc. During mediation, you should request information to be produced in native file format so that you may capture that all-important metadata.

Spoliation

Don't be overly concerned about the destruction of or manipulation of ESMI. The failure to produce ESMI can lead to very severe consequences for the culprit. These consequences may include:

- Malpractice
- Imposition of court sanctions
- Loss of an otherwise winnable case
- Summary judgment in your favor
- Disciplinary action

In efforts to punctuate the severity of spoliation of evidence, there are two landmark decisions I'd like you to review:

1. Coleman (Parent) Holdings, Inc. v. Morgan Stanley & Co., Inc., 2005 WL 67071 (Fla. Cir. Ct. Mar. 1, 2005), rev'd on other grounds, 955 So.2d 1124 (Fla. 4th CA 2007), and
2. Zubulake v. UBS Warburg, LLC, 229 F.R.D. 422 (D.N.Y. 2004).

In these decisions, the court issued adverse inference instructions for spoliation of evidence. As a result, the jury in the Morgan Stanley case returned with a $1.4 billion verdict; and the jury in Zubulake returned with a $29 million verdict.

*Note: Spoliation of evidence is the intentional or negligent withholding, hiding, altering, or destroying of evidence relevant to a legal proceeding. See, *Wikipedia.org*.

Federal and State Rules Relating to ESMI

On December 1, 2006, changes relating to electronically stored information (ESMI) in the Federal Rules of Civil Procedure metastasized. The changes affected Rules 16, 26, 33, 34, 37, 45 and Form 35 and provided mandates to the preservation, discoverability, production, accessibility, and costs associated with ESMI. Federal courts have issued local rules of practice and guidelines regarding ESMI. Visit www.elawexchange.com under the section entitled "Leading Decisions and Fed. Rules" for a more comprehensive look at the framework for the discovery of electronic data.

For an up-to-date listing of state-by-state electronic discovery case decisions and procedural rules, visit www.elawexchange.com for online access. And, don't forget to check your state's court rules in relation to electronic discovery and evidence!

CHAPTER 3

Forms, Types, and Storage of ESMI

Increasing volumes of electronically stored information (ESI), evolving e-discovery case law, the automation of legal processes, changing ESI protocols, and harsher judicial sanctions have fueled the need for electronically stored medical information (ESMI). In response to this trend, a growing number of healthcare professionals are investing in consultative e-discovery talent, focusing on the healthcare industry, to ensure litigation readiness.

There are many different forms of electronically stored information (ESMI) that should be considered in your quest to uncover relevant evidence. Principal "forms" that should be considered when discussing the disclosure of ESMI should include:

- Native File
- Database
- Spreadsheet
- Image
- ASCII, TEXT, and Conversion Formats, i.e., .PDF and .TIFF
- Video and Audio
- Paper
- ALS and Online ESMI Repository

Also, there are different "types" of ESMI, as well, including:

- E-mail
- Word Processing Documents
- Spreadsheets
- Voicemail messages and files
- Backup email files
- Deleted Emails
- Data files
- Program files
- Backup Archival Tapes
- Temporary files
- System History Files

*Note: Request the forms of ESMI that are most advantageous to your needs, i.e., native file format to view hidden metadata.

Another important topic of consideration should concern the possible storage media, devices, and locations of ESMI. Understanding these areas will not only help you pinpoint the discovery of relevant ESMI, but also the production of ESMI.

Storage Media

Storage media is used to store data from an electronic device. These storage devices could include a floppy disc, hard drive, thumb drive, CD-ROM, DVD, Blu-ray Disk, Smart Card, and Microfilm/Microfiche.

Storage Devices

Storage devices use the storage media discussed above. The storage devices are the places where the storage media must be placed in efforts to see, hear and enjoy the data. Some of the most common storage devices include a mainframe computer, printer, copier, personal computer, laptop, PDA, cell phone, voice mail, pager, and scanner.

Just think of the storage device as the place where that DVD or thumb drive needs to be placed in order to view the data once you receive it from the producing party.

Storage Locations

The location is the place where the actual "physical" data can be found. This is one of the most important challenges of uncovering relevant electronic data, which is why you will need to conduct an Electronic Discovery Identification and Preservation Questionnaire, which is designed to help identify, preserve and collect electronically stored information for discovery. Storage locations may include Service Providers for the Internet, Satellite, Pagers, Cellular phones, Financial Institutions / Credit Card Issuers, Credit Bureau Repositories, Cable Service Providers, as well as Internet Storage Locations such as the World Wide Web, chat rooms, newsgroups, Facebook, LinkedIn, Cache files, etc.

The purpose of the Electronic Discovery Identification and Preservation Questionnaire is for you to gain an understanding of the producing party's computer system so that you have a working knowledge of how their ESMI is created, stored, and retained. Remember the words "native file format" mentioned at the top of the chapter? Well, that simply means the way that a data file is "reasonably usable" or "ordinarily maintained". That would mean that the data format is proprietary and not transferrable unless a conversion software is used.

Example: Microsoft Excel is saved in proprietary format with the file extension .XLS. In Excel, you can open, modify, and save any changes to the file. If you wanted to use the same file in Lotus 1-2-3, then, a conversion process would need to be performed on the .XLS file. The conversion process may not accurately convert the file in the new Lotus format because metadata may be lost inadvertently.

Note: Courts have held that a producing party should provide electronic discovery in its native file format. The scrubbing or erasing metadata from native files without agreement of the requesting party is sanctionable conduct. Producing ESMI in native file format allows a party to view the original document including any metadata and tracked changes. The failure to ask for "metadata" in the original request may preclude later discovery of the all-important hidden data. And, courts have consistently held that disclosure in a .TIFF or .PDF format, as opposed to a "native file" format is unusable, notwithstanding a party's ability to redact and Bates-stamp .TIFF images.

Some Important Rules You Can Use

As previously mentioned, on December 1, 2006, changes relating to the preservation, discoverability, production, accessibility, and costs associated with electronically stored information (ESI) took effect in the Federal Rules of Civil Procedure. These changes will impact most cases in federal court and your state court may have changes that will mirror the federal changes.

We will not attempt to peruse every nook and cranny of the rules, state or federal, but will highlight some important decisions relating to the discoverability of ESI to give you a working knowledge of their importance, and allow you the opportunity to speak intelligently at your upcoming Rule 26(f) "Meet and Confer" conference or your state level Case Management Conference in regards to the request and production of electronically stored information.

Rules Requiring Cooperation Between Parties

Federal Rules of Civil Procedure 16(a): The court may order a pretrial conference of all parties for such purposes as:

- Expediting disposition
- Establishing early and continuing control of a case
- Discourage wasteful pretrial activities
- Improve the quality through more thorough preparation
- Facilitation of settlement

Federal Rules of Civil Procedure 26(a)(1): Parties must, without awaiting discovery request, disclose to other parties:

- Witnesses who may have discoverable information and description and location of ESI relevant to the case
- Computation of each category of damages claimed and make evidentiary material available for inspection and copying, unless privileged or protected from disclosure

Federal Rules of Civil Procedure 26(b)(2)(C): Provides the Courts the inherent authority to limit discovery *sua sponte* or on motion if:

- Requests are unreasonably cumulative or duplicative
- Requests are obtainable from more convenient, less burdensome or inexpensive source
- A party has had plenty of opportunity to obtain information during action, and burden or expense of proposed discovery outweighs likely benefit in light of case needs, amount in controversy, parties' resources, importance of issues and of discovery to those issues

Federal Rules of Civil Procedure 26(f): Conference Planning Obligations aka "Meet and Confer". The parties must meet as soon as practicable to:

- Consider possibilities for settlement/resolution
- Arrange disclosures required by Rule 26(a)(1)
- Discuss issues about preserving ESI
- Disclose custodian name and discoverable data sources
- Develop a discovery plan and written report

Federal Rules of Civil Procedure 26(g): Certification. Every disclosure and discovery request, response, or objection must be signed by at least one attorney of record certifying the disclosure is complete and correct to best of their knowledge, information and belief formed after:

- Reasonable inquiry that the disclosures were complete and correct at the time made
- Discovery requests and responses are consistent with existing law
- Not interposed for improper purpose
- Neither unreasonable nor unduly burdensome or expensive in light of case needs, amount in controversy, and importance of issues at stake

Important ESI Case Law and Legal Hold

In order to truly understand the importance and relevance of ESI case law, you must first understand the concept of the "**litigation hold**" or "**legal hold**". Remember, the litigation hold, or legal hold is one of the most important, if not **the** most important part of the entire litigation. This directive is an ongoing process to preserve electronically stored information, documents, or physical evidence pertaining to "reasonably anticipated" litigation. If you are a pro se litigant, you would not issue a legal hold per se, but would issue a "**Data Preservation Notice or Request**" to opposing counsel about what has been preserved, what you would like preserved, and request his or her reasonable input as to whether other ESI needs to be preserved.

1. Zubulake v. UBS Warbug, LLC, 220 F.R.D. 212, 218 (S.D.N.Y. 2003) (Scheindlin, S.)("[o]nce a party reasonably anticipates litigation, it must suspend its routine document retention/destruction policy and put in place a legal hold to ensure the preservation of relevant documents").

2. Pension Comm. Of the Univ. of Montreal Pension Plan v. Banc of Am. Secs, LLC, No. 05-9016, 2010 U.S. Dist. LEXIS 4546 (S.D.N.Y. Jan. 15, 2010), as corrected, Docket #358 (May 28, 2010)("[a] plaintiff's duty is more often triggered before litigation commences, in large part because plaintiffs control the timing of litigation").

3. <u>Victor Stanley, Inc. v. Creative Pipe, Inc. "Victor Stanley II"</u>, U.S. Dist. LEXIS 93644 (D. Md. Sept. 9, 2010), where U.S. District Judge Paul W. Grimm provided counsel with "an analytical framework that may enable them to resolve preservation/spoliation issues with a greater level of comfort that their actions will not expose them to disproportionate costs or unpredictable outcomes of spoliation motions." The court's discussion also included numerous key points and a "Law of Spoliation" framework that outlines the scope of duty to preserve among other culpability and prejudice requirements in each of the federal circuits.

Depending on the common law of your jurisdiction, the duty to preserve relevant evidence arises when litigation is "reasonably anticipated"; "pending, imminent, reasonably foreseeable"; "pending or impending". Again, consult Judge Grimm's "Law of Spoliation" framework for guidance on what the common law of your jurisdiction may be with respect to preservation of evidence.

One final caveat: A document retention policy that repeatedly and automatically destroys electronically stored information on a consistent and timely schedule without any regards to any legal hold directive will face severe consequences if the policy is not modified to suspend the destruction once litigation is reasonably anticipated.

Sounds serious, huh? Well, it is! Failure to have an e-discovery litigation readiness program in place can and will lead to severe consequences for the healthcare professional. Let's take a look at how to request ESMI.

CHAPTER 4

Requesting Electronically Stored Medical Information

When requesting ESMI in discovery, the first step is to determine the specific, relevant case information you want from the responding side.

Your electronic information objectives should focus on how the responding side used computers or EMR System to generate data or documents during the events in question.

If health information was requested from a hospital then you have to determine whether or not their information systems captured the different steps in treating and providing care to the patient. Finally, if you wanted to determine if a person was blind copied on an electronic message, then electronic messaging data would be requested thus allowing you to view the e-mail and metadata.

When requesting discovery, it is important to target ESMI responsive to your claims. This may include e-mail, word processing files, databases, Internet history files, calendars, and schedules—virtually any ESMI. In addition, you will need to focus on ESMI storage devices (computers, PDA's, cellular phones, etc.), storage media (hard drives, backup tapes, pen drives, etc.,) and the storage locations (home offices, central servers, etc.).

Nature of Claims and Defenses

The nature of the case, claims and defenses, and defenses, and factual issues will define the type and source of ESMI that you will be seeking. The Federal Rules of Civil Procedure directives, and generally state court procedural rules, revolve around the claims and defenses of a specific case.

In addition, requesting excessive data would increase the burden on the producing and requesting party to conduct a meaningful review of the data. Be prepared for the producing party to attempt to limit your request by:

- Arguing that the information sought is not relevant to the claims or defenses;
- Offering an alternative procedure for locating and producing records that you are seeking, such as proposing a list of keywords to be used

in conducting searches or a list of directories or servers to be searched;

- Limit your searches of e-mail or other electronic information to specific personnel or date ranges; and
- Submitting a substantial cost estimate and extended schedule for screening and production of electronic information.

If that should happen, and it most certainly will, there are techniques that can be deployed to minimize the effect of the above challenges and limit the amount of ESMI to be produced, reduce costs, and narrow the scope of discovery.

One thing I would do is **narrow the subject matter of the request to the specific claims or defenses of the case**. If your case is in regards to storage of ESMI that had occurred on a specific date, narrow the production request to the date that the input of the medical data was to have occurred.

If there was a specific individual who had claimed to have input data on behalf of a hospital or clinic, then, **limit the scope of discovery to that specific individual**.

Don't forget to **request load files with metadata**! If you are collecting data in an electronic format, you will need to request metadata to be included so that you can determine when the file was created, by whom, and where.

Finally, **reach an agreement with opposing counsel as to what ESMI is "not reasonably accessible".** By doing so, you take away that protection and have an agreement in writing as to what ESMI will and will not be produced.

CHAPTER 5

"MEET AND CONFER" PLANNING GUIDE

Federal Rules of Civil Procedure 26(f) requires parties in litigation to "...confer as soon as practicable...[and to]...state the parties' views and proposals on...any issues about disclosure or discovery of electronically stored information..." You need to be sure that you properly handle this "meet-and-confer" session about electronically stored medical information in order to put yourself in position to effectively negotiate a resolution on the matter at hand. Let's face it, approximately 95% of all cases in litigation do not make it to trial. They are settled using some form of ADR (Alternative Dispute Resolution), i.e., mediation, arbitration, conciliation, negotiation. In fact, most state and federal local rules require that cases be referred to mediation or arbitration, before formal litigation. And, Rule 68 of the Federal Rules of Civil Procedure, enacted in 1938, and state counterparts, give the party who is defending a claim the opportunity to settle by making a formal offer of judgment.

The party who rejects the settlement offer is liable for sanctions if final judgment is not "more favorable" than the settlement offer.

If the amount of any final judgment is less than the settlement offer, after monetary calculations, the prevailing party is required to pay all "costs incurred after the making of the offer." So, as you can see, you should always be thinking about putting yourself in the best possible position for settlement during the discovery process. With that being said, let's talk about the seven deadly sins of the Rule 26(f) "meet-and-confer" and how to minimize e-discovery costs and risks to make sure you will be able to get the data you need from the opposition.

Seven Deadly Sins

Deadly Sin #1: Failure to Set the Agenda. Set the agenda means to come prepared to the Rule 26(f) conference and make sure the opponent is prepared as well. You can accomplish this by sending a "Data Preservation Letter" early in the litigation process. The letter will intimate what you expect to accomplish at the conference, what information you will bring to the conference, and what information you expect from the opposition.

Deadly Sin #2: Failure to Manage Preservation. Again, be sure to communicate what you need as far as data in the "Data Preservation Letter". Disclose your preservation decisions early on and be prepared to explain why you have chosen to do so. Demand the same from your opponent. Their data is part of your case and you need to make sure it is secured.

Deadly Sin #3: Failure to Corral E-Discovery and Limit and Phase E-Discovery. Remember, e-discovery is determined by the importance of the data to the case, and the dollar value in proportion to the case. Present a sensible plan to corral the important data. Only a handful of documents are likely to be used at trial, mediation or arbitration. Suggest starting with two or three key employees and build from there. If the question is in regards to electronic medical records, start with the names of the personnel responsible for data entry and build from there. Reach agreement on a flexible, rolling e-discovery plan for the continued production of documents as you uncover additional parties that may have input data for the hospital or healthcare agency.

Deadly Sin #4: Failure to Set Search Expectations. Make sure that you insist on search quality and demonstrable, statistically valid recall. High recall means the search is pulling most, if not all, the responsive documents. Don't let the opposition test for precision and not test for recall. In a medical malpractice case, you will encounter questions of precision and recall, and if you are a paralegal or hospital administrator working on a large scale e-discovery case, contact me for further information on precision and recall.

Deadly Sin #5: Failure to Specify the Production Format. Establish the production format in your "Request for Production of Documents". Included in this e-book is a format on how to request documents to include load files with metadata. If a third party vendor is to be used, get the vendor's delivery specifications and provide it early to the opposition. Don't let the opposition decide what format is reasonably useable for the case.

Deadly Sin #6: Failure to Protect Against Privilege Waiver from Inadvertent Production. Let's face it...mistakes happen. And, they will happen during the production of documents. If you are a paralegal working a large scale e-discovery case, be sure to get the entry of a court order, under Federal Rules of Evidence 502, protecting you against inadvertent disclosure of privileged documents and providing that any determination of non-waiver arising from an inadvertent production is also binding on state court proceedings.

Negotiate a written protocol with the opposition as to the procedures to be followed if a privileged document is discovered to have been inadvertently produced.

Deadly Sin #7: Failure to Document. If at all possible, hire a mediator to facilitate any e-discovery disputes. That way, the mediator can draft a "Memorandum of Understanding" and memorialize the conference as you would a settlement agreement or contract. Mediation of ESI disputes is a growing field in the world of e-discovery as data is becoming more abundant. Don't let what you have accomplished at the Rule 26(f) get lost along the road to success.

The simple way to ensure that your healthcare organization does not violate any of the sins is to engage a consultant in efforts to educate your organization as follows:

- *ESMI Education*: Despite the growing importance of technology in the healthcare industry, many doctors and healthcare executives lack an understanding of the complexities of e-discovery and the technicalities required to collect, process and review electronic data.

- *Technology Expertise*: E-Discovery practitioners leverage technology to help clients streamline workloads and mitigate the risks and expense associated with e-discovery in the healthcare context.
- *Litigation Readiness*: Healthcare organizations that implement a litigation readiness plan can minimize the costs of e-discovery and reduce response time in the event of litigation. E-discovery professionals can help a healthcare organization develop a strategy for preserving relevant data and assist clients in drafting, implementing and complying with litigation holds and preservation orders.
- *Data Collection and Review*: The collection and review stages of e-discovery are often the most costly and labor-intensive. E-discovery consultants guide healthcare professionals through the critical decision-making process of key word or contextual-based searching and streamline the review process to avoid mistakes and minimize expense.
- *Risk Management*: Healthcare organizations are subject to heavy sanctions for litigation abuses and a failure to comply with e-discovery rules. E-discovery consultants help develop the best

practices and defensible discovery solutions that minimize the risk and cost of e-discovery.

- _Records-Retention Protocols_: Managing volumes of ESMI begins with the creation of an effective records-management policy. E-discovery consultants will consult with healthcare professionals in designing records-retention protocols that comply with legal and regulatory retention mandates and meet the needs of the healthcare organization.

As the need for ESMI matures, healthcare organizations will to become acquainted with the legal knowledge, technological know-how, management expertise, and innovative thinking to ensure that their organization is e-discovery compliant in the event that litigation becomes imminent or impending.

Chapter 6
Rule 26(f) Conference Preparation

Okay, you've filed an answer to the complaint, requested your first set of interrogatories, ESMI interrogatories, expert witness interrogatories, and request for production of documents to include load files with metadata. Now, you should be prepared to meet with the opposing party and speak intelligently about the nature and extent of potentially relevant ESMI. We will examine some questions that should be addressed and illuminate the reasons why these questions should be asked and answered, BEFORE the Rule 26(f) Conference:

1. What are the issues in the case? The parties should be on the page as to what the issues are so that there are no objections as to the preservation and production of relevant ESMI.
2. Who are the key players in the case? Identifying the key custodians is critical to uncovering who have relevant ESMI.
3. Who are the persons most knowledgeable about ESMI systems? You will need to communicate with someone who can describe the network infrastructure and organization of ESMI, including locations of user files and storage areas, as well as

file servers, email servers, application servers, and web servers.

4. What events and intervals are relevant? Narrowing down the relevant time frame is essential to narrowing the scope of relevant ESMI.

5. When did preservation duties and privileges attach? You want to investigate and find out whether a formal Litigation Hold has been implemented. Remember, the party initiating the litigation has a duty to preserve ESMI much earlier than the responding party.

6. What steps have been or will be taken to preserve ESMI? In addition to uncovering whether a formal Litigation Hold has been implemented, you will also want to know whether there is a written records retention/destruction policy, and if so, has the data destruction and auto-deletion policies have been suspended.

7. What third parties hold information that must be preserved, and who will notify them? This is especially important in medical malpractice litigation where EHR/EMR will be involved. The electronic medical records' database would be subject to discovery.

8. What forms of production are offered or sough? Will the opposing party produce the documents in

native file format? .TIFF? Will the data be provided on a CD-ROM? Flash drive? Paper format?

9. What ESMI will be claimed as not reasonably accessible, and on what basis? This is an important inquiry because you can narrow your scope of what ESMI is relevant and if the other side objects, you can ask why and have a meeting of the minds to ascertain what is reasonably accessible and what is not.

10. When is the next Rule 26(f) Conference (because you will need to do this more than once).

For somewhat different approaches to the E-Discovery topics to be addressed at a Rule 26(f) Conference, be sure to visit the discussion of Magistrate Judge Paul W. Grimm at: www.mdd.uscourts.gov/news/news/ESIProtocol.pdf.

Finally, here are more questions that will help punctuate the importance of proper Rule 26(f) preparation:

1. What are the issues in the case?
2. Who are the key players in the case?
3. Who are the persons most knowledgeable about EHR/EMR systems?

4. What events and intervals are relevant?

5. When did preservation duties and privileges attach?

6. What steps have been or will be taken to preserve ESMI?

7. Has a Litigation Hold taken place?   If so, when?

8. What third parties hold information that must be preserved, and who will notify them?

9. What metadata is relevant, and how will it be preserved, extracted and produced?

10.   What are the data retention policies and practices?

11.   What are the backup practices, and what tape archives exist?

12.   Are there legacy systems to be addressed?

13.   How will the parties handle voice mail, instant messaging and other challenging ESMI?

14.   Is there a preservation duty going forward, and how will it be met?

15.   Is a preservation or protective order needed?

16.   Will paper documents be scanned, at what resolution and with what OCR and metadata?

17.   What search techniques will be used to identify responsive or privileged ESMI?

18.   What forms of production are offered or sought?

19.   Will single or multi-page .TIFF;s, .PDF's or other image formats be produced?

20.   Will load files accompany document images, and how will they be populated?

21.   Will there be a need for native file production? Quasi-native production?

22.   On what media will ESI be delivered? Optical disks? External drives? Thumb drives?

23.   How will we handle inadvertent production of privileged ESI?

24.   How will we protect trade secrets and other confidential information in the ESMI?

25.   How do we resolve questions about printouts before their use in deposition or at trial?

26.   How will we handle authentication of the native ESI used in deposition or trial?

27.   Who will serve as liaisons or coordinators for each side on ESMI issues?

28.   Will technical assistants be permitted to communicate directly?

29.   Is there a need for an E-Discovery Special Master or Mediator?

30.   Can any costs be shared or shifted by agreement?

31.   How much time is required to identify, collect, process, review, redact, and produce ESMI?

Use the enclosed 101 tips as a guide to help you stay abreast of what you need to become and remain e-discovery compliant in your healthcare organization.

ACKNOWLEDGEMENTS

1. Arkfeld's Best Practices Guide for Electronic Discovery and Evidence, by Michael R. Arkfeld

2. "Bitter Pill" series of articles in TIME Magazine 2013, by Steven Brill

3. GP SOLO, A Publication of the American Bar Association, "How Technology Is Changing the Practice of Law", by Blair Janis, JD

4. "An Update From GDC, August 2012", Electronic Discovery in Healthcare Litigation, by Garson DeCorato & Cohen, LLP, Attorneys at Law

5. Bill Hamilton's "Seven Deadly Sins of the Rule 26(f) Conference", by William H. Hamilton, Dean of Graduate Studies, Bryan University, E-Discovery Project Management

6. "Medical Deficit Disorder", by Anthony Johnson

7. "Breaking Into E-Discovery", by Sally A. Kane

101 Tips for the Healthcare Professional

FORWARD

"Many cases that should involve electronic documents, and therefore e-discovery, end up in courtrooms with nothing but boxes of paper and binders. Here's the scary reason behind that reality: Most lawyers, even those who use a range of technology every day, are still uncomfortable dealing with electronic documents in discovery. Hence, there is often a tacit or even an explicit agreement between opposing counsels of the "don't ask for e-documents and I won't either" type. The worst part is that generally these lawyers are convinced they are helping their clients by saving them money and hassle. In most cases, the opposite is the truth." – Atty Dominic Jaar

Source:

www.americanbar.org/publications/law_practice_home/law_practice_archive/LPM_Magazine_Articles_v35_IS2_pg50.html

"Some trial attorneys, with or without the permission of their clients, go so far as to enter into secret agreements with each other to ignore the [ESI] world" -- Atty Ralph Losey

Source:
HTTP://E-DISCOVERYTEAM.COM/SCHOOL/PLATO%E2%80%99S-CAVE-WHY-MOST-LAWYERS-LOVE-PAPER-AND-HATE-E-DISCOVERY-AND-WHAT-THIS-MEANS-TO-THE-FUTURE-OF-LEGAL-EDUCATION/

"...[e-Discovery is] so new that virtually no one knows how to do it. As a result most lawyers do their best to avoid it, and when they cannot, they hire outside experts to tell them what to do. Or, worse yet, they blunder through blindly on their own and mess up at their client's expense."
-- Atty Ralph Losey

Source:

http://e-discoveryteam.com/2011/01/09/the-law-firm-apprenticeship-tradition-and-why-most-lawyers-are-still-untrained-in-e-discovery/

TIP #1

To save yourself and your office staff time and money -- seek out and retain the services of a law firm or an attorney who is comfortable, knowledgeable, and has proven experience with e-Discovery because many law schools do not teach this subject in law school.

TIP #2

Knowledge is Power: Therefore, if you are party to a lawsuit and the opposing counsel has and uses e-Discovery and your legal representative doesn't -- then guess what? Right, you're already behind the power curve.

TIP #3

Create and store your medical records in a way that allows you and / or your staff to easily preserve and retrieve potentially relevant data in the event of litigation and in compliance with both state and federal ediscovery rules.

TIP #4

As a result of a recent New York appellate court ruling that "the party producing the data is the one that should bear the costs" -- there now exists the potential for even more e-Discovery requests to be made by an aggressive plaintiff attorney that you may face.

TIP #5

Identify and know who is a "custodian" of the medical records in your office practice and the different locations where these records are kept and maintained.

TIP #6

Set up a separate computer server dedicated to storing all relevant data related to litigation so that you can quickly respond and readily produce any required records.

TIP #7

Create and map all electronic storage devices and records management data systems that are used in your office practice prior to being involved in a litigation matter.

TIP #8

Train your office staff and be proactive so that they know what to do and understand the process in the event of receiving an e-Discovery request or litigation hold.

TIP #9

If you use a mobile device to interact with your patients (i.e. charting patient data) -- remember that even if you have lost your cellphone, tablet, or laptop computer -- the data still exists somewhere on a computer server and could be potentially discoverable.

TIP #10

Healthcare providers must know where the data is located so that they can take steps to preserve it in the event of litigation.

TIP #11

Healthcare providers need to be aware of other "custodians" (i.e. medical residents, medical students, committees, other allied health professionals, etc) who may be creating and storing data relevant to their patient remotely that does not get entered into the hospital EMR system.

TIP #12

Raw data that is created by a third-party using proprietary software may not be accessible to a plaintiff or defense attorney to help defend a healthcare provider involved in a lawsuit.

TIP #13

The more information that is potentially stored on any device the greater the risk of it being discoverable and made available to the opposing counsel -- therefore, seek to reduce the amount of all unnecessary information in a patient record.

TIP #14

Be sure to update you paper and electronic records retention policy so that it parallels with your e-Discovery preparation and legal hold training / plans.

TIP #15

Be aware that litigation hold includes all paging, billing, email, systems as well as the usual medical records that are created by computer, on a mobile device, tablet, cellphone, etc.

TIP #16

Healthcare providers need to remember that an audit trail can be created that reveals via time-data stamp everything that occurs to an electronically stored file.

TIP #17

Check with a local healthcare atty to see if you are protected in the event of inadvertently releasing protected information pursuant to your attempt to fulfill an e-Discovery request.

TIP #18

Check with your local healthcare atty to see what the retention policy is on emails, text messages, and faxed documents that may be incidental but not directly related to the care of a patient -- you want to know if and when these "potentially relevant" items should be saved.

TIP #19

Be aware of any potential state law requirements that certain patient-related records be kept and maintained according to a forthcoming uniformity standard, be interchangeable, or have a certain ease of use.

TIP #20

Take a proactive stance and look for ways to decrease your potential e-discovery costs before litigation occurs.

TIP #21

Read, understand, and research the case law, court procedural rules, and legal rules in your state regarding e-Discovery.

TIP #22

The increased number of ICD-10 diagnostic codes will increase the range, scope, and availability of e-Discovery tools that could be used in a litigation matter.

TIP #23

Anticipate potential litigation and create a standardized process with policies and procedures that your office will use in **the** event of receiving an e-Discovery request or litigation hold notice.

TIP #24

Remember that often, there may exist a lot more information about a given patient than what the doctor may see when they pull up the patient's chart on a computer screen.

TIP #25

Request your atty conduct an audit trail to verify and authenticate the integrity, chronology, and the reliability of the electronic medical records concerning the care, events, treatments, outcome, and results of a patient that could be used in a legal matter.

TIP #26

Consider the Cost of Lost Time per Year to your practice:

Assume busy practice, 4 satellite offices, 50 employees, 16 Litigation Hold Matters, Employees per Matter, Employee hours spent per year = 240, gives Cost of Lost Time per year of $12,528.

TIP #27

Metadata is defined as "data about the data" and the best example is the date-time-stamp that's electronically created each time a healthcare provider uses his security access card to enter the hospital, logs onto the hospital computer, or dictates a radiology report.

TIP #28

Understand that metadata can disclose what time a document was created, who created it, when it was viewed, and who logged in to access the document, if the document was altered, modified, or changed from its original form.

TIP #29

Think of e-Discovery as "CSI on steroids" when it comes to looking at your electronic medical records and information about your patient.

TIP #30

Check with your medical liability insurance carrier to see if they offer any premium discounts because you utilize electronic medical records in your practice.

TIP #31

Schedule your hospital CIO to speak to the Medical Staff about e-Discovery and its impact on your practice at least once a year.

TIP #32

Take a photo of each employee holding their own personal portable devices (name, model, brand) to assist you in creating a retention policy, ESI record keeping, and maintaining track of the potential sources of electronic medical data.

TIP #33

There are over twenty-one data types (i.e. text msg, photo, cellphone call, landline phone call, voicemail, video camera, digital webcam, fax, email, instagram, twitter, Excel spreadsheet, slideshow, Word document, security access badge, debit card, credit card, car transponder, pager, laptop computer, desk computer, tablet, pop-up warnings, etc.

TIP #34

Read the multiple published legal opinions Zubulake v UBS Warburg holding that "[b]road electronic discovery is a cornerstone of the litigation process contemplated by the Federal Rules of Civil Procedure."

TIP #35

Know the legal rules and the case law that pertains to your practice location, including the procedural court rules.

TIP #36

Try to determine and to narrow the scope of any potential e-Discovery request as early as possible in the litigation process.

TIP #37

Understand that the scope of an e-Discovery request could include providing e-mails, voice mail, medical records, billing and reimbursement information, payroll and marketing data, and credit card transactions and where this information is stored.

TIP #38

Penalties that physicians could face due to failure to comply with e-Discovery requests include having to "pay the opponent's discovery and attorney fees", lost opportunity to "make certain arguments to a jury with respect to missing evidence" and dismissal of their case.

TIP #39

Remember that an audit trail conducted by a computer forensic specialist can determine who, when, where, and how an electronically stored record was accessed and sometime, why the record was accessed.

TIP #40

If you are in litigation, try to avoid the court imposing an adverse inference instruction on you and understand why this should be avoided at all costs.

TIP #41

If in litigation or litigation is eminent, ask your atty how to help you best prevent the court from issuing an adverse inference instruction against you.

TIP #42

Ask your professional liability insurance carrier how many cases they settled on behalf of their physician policyholders since the implementation of e-Discovery changes took place effective 1 Dec 2006.

TIP #43

Of those cases settled favorably on behalf of their policyholders, how many of them did your professional liability insurance carrier advantageously use e-Discovery?

TIP #44

If you atty does not use e-Discovery, then immediately hire another one who does.

TIP #45

Ask your atty to send you a copy of the scheduling order that is related to the provisions for disclosure or discovery of electronically stored information.

TIP #46

Since ESI is considered "reasonably accessible" and "not reasonably accessible", the physician should be aware of the importance to preserve inaccessible ESI.

TIP #47

If in litigation, be sure your atty asks for a court order that protects you and your staff in the event of producing and releasing protected information and documents by mistake pursuant to a discovery request.

TIP #48

Ask your hospital IT staff and/or Hospital Atty to walk you through their Litigation hold procedure and understand what specific duties and responsibilities may be required of you.

TIP #49

Ask your hospital IT staff and CEO/Admin when was the last time and how often they upgraded or improved the security of ESI related to the hospital network.

TIP #50

Ask the hospital CEO to disclose the IT budget and IT staffing since 1 Dec 2006 and to explain if and why there is any consistent reduction in these numbers given the importance of ESI.

TIP #51

Write a letter to the hospital CEO expressing your concern and objection to any reduced IT budget and staffing -- this could provide some degree of protection in the event you are named with the hospital as a co-Defendant in future litigation.

TIP #52

Annually review your document retention policy in light of new court cases or changes in the law that become effective within the next 6-12 months.

TIP #53

Request/invite an outside ESI consultant to conduct an inspection of your office and computer system to assist you with preparing, developing, and planning for a litigation hold or e-Discovery request.

TIP #54

Ask the hospital to provide a representative from the legal, IT, HR, Risk Management, Compliance, Operations departments to host a panel discussion for the medical staff at their Quarterly Medical Staff meeting.

TIP #55

Appoint someone in your office-based practice and your hospital-based practice to handle ESI litigation matters -- preferably someone who has an interested in this area.

TIP #56

Know what the statute of limitations and records retention laws are for your state -- Under 45 CFR Section 164.530(j), HIPAA requires medical records to be maintained for six years.

TIP #57

E-discovery related to employment litigation may require swifter action since the Fair labor Standards Act and the Equal Pay Act do not require companies to retain employment records for more than three years.

TIP #58

Create your own timeline of events related to the case in order to assist your legal defense team.

TIP #59

Prepare and update your professional resume, including a list of the past two years of CME hours earned.

TIP #60

Demonstrate that your practice of medicine is in conformance with your employment contract or shareholder agreement as well as in accordance with certain policies, procedures, criteria, and standards established by a recognized national professional healthcare organization and / or entity that is particular to your specialty.

TIP #61

Spoliation and tampering with evidence and the medical records raises a red flag that can backfire and lead to a dismissal of your case and any evidence that is used to support your position.

TIP #62

Be aware that a printed copy of a document may be fundamentally different than the electronic record as it is stored on a computer server.

TIP #63

There are two kinds of meta-data: application metadata and system metadata. Both of which can change over time due to the software and the operating system on the computer.

TIP #64

The three P's of eDiscovery are: people, processes, and proportionality. If people understand the process, then they can use technology and the tools of eDiscovery to reduce their overall litigation costs.

TIP #65

The producing party normally bears the costs of discovery -- and the requesting party can gain leverage during litigation by forcing or threatening to force the producing party to incur high discovery costs.

TIP #66

There may be a time lag or difference in the time that a procedure was actually performed and the time-stamp that is created in the EMR when the information about the procedure was physically entered into the computer system.

TIP #67

If the law firm is using predictive coding software as an e-Discovery tool, be sure that the senior attorney who has first-hand knowledge of all the facts and the legal theory and strategy of the case is the one who trains the predictive coding software platform. Otherwise, a junior associate with limited legal skills and experience may inadvertently fail to properly train the software and thus it will miss important responsive documents.

This could result in additional legal costs, sanctions and possibly losing the case.

TIP #68

The use of eDiscovery not only provides leverage but it also directly impacts the overall litigation costs and budget of the litigants and can influence the decision-makers during settlement negotiations.

TIP #69

Considering the overall litigation costs and the damages being sought, the effective use of eDiscovery can help a party determine whether they should proceed with filing a complaint, whether it would be prudent to be more aggressive and proceed with more directed discovery, or whether it would be best to settle a given legal matter.

TIP #70

Ask your atty if they are personally familiar with and have recently read the e-discovery obligations that are required by your jurisdiction's Local Rules of Court. If so, then request that the atty provide you with a copy of what they read. If they have no personal knowledge and / or have not read it, then hire another atty.

TIP #71

Be proactive about eDiscovery -- do not let the knowledge deficit that lawyers, law firms, and judges have about eDiscovery hurt you or your case.

TIP #72

Organize and present the most relevant important documents and information first to help your atty most efficiently review, determine, and prepare for the most cost-effective way to handle the legal matter.

TIP #73

Remember that eDiscovery lives at the intersection of law and technology — therefore, if your atty is not using the best technology available to help you win your case, can you afford to take that risk? It's almost like practicing medicine before the use of CT scanning.

TIP #74

Relevant case law as well as local, state, and federal rules dictate the rules related to eDiscovery in a given jurisdiction -- however, these rules may vary significantly by jurisdiction.

TIP #75

Court rules targeting e-discovery have already been enacted in more than thirty states -- thus it would behoove healthcare providers to become familiar with them.

TIP #76

In preparation of your atty defending you or pursuing e-Discovery as part of your legal strategy, be sure to <u>first</u> -- get your own house in order.

TIP #77

Avoid the trap of destroying potentially relevant electronically stored information and thinking that your document retention policy will protect you from any adverse outcome pursuant to a litigation hold notice.

TIP #78

Create an "ESI DOCUMENT RETENTION POLICY CHECKLIST" that is specific for your practice.

TIP #79

Create a "ESI LITIGATION HOLD CHECKLIST" that is specific for your practice.

TIP #80

Create an "INITIAL E-DISCOVERY CHECKLIST" that is specific for your practice.

TIP #81

Hospitals that ignore eDiscovery rules can face severe sanctions -- see Report and Recommendation (Report) on a motion for sanctions alleging spoliation of medical records, in U.S. ex. rel. Elin Baklid-Kunz v. Halifax Hospital Medical Center et. al.

TIP #82

Clients may complain about the exorbitant costs of eDiscovery – however, the evidentiary and financial costs due to spoliation can be much more severe and devastating.

TIP #83

It's important that a good working relationship exists between the healthcare provider, his counsel, and the opposing counsel to minimize the overall costs due to e-Discovery.

TIP #84

Create a data map of your practice --
which may be no more than 2-3 page
summary of your electronic and paper
data storage systems.

TIP #85

Healthcare providers involved in a legal
malpractice claim should consider asking
for a copy of the attorney's file to see if
and how e-Discovery was (or was not)
advantageously used to help them.

TIP #86

Information stored on a hospital EMR
system (today) may not look the same on
either the computer monitor or the paper
record that was used then (i.e. the date of

an alleged medical malpractice event four years ago) due to software upgrades during the interim.

TIP #87

Defendant healthcare providers involved in frivolous lawsuits should consider seeking recovery of e-Discovery costs pursuant to "offers of judgment" -- see Federal Rule of Civil Procedure 68.

TIP #88

Certain litigation expenses may qualify as "taxable costs" -- see 28 U.S.C. §1920

TIP #89

If a producing party converts their medical data and information into a TIFF format that has metadata before transferring it to a review platform" then this results in an "ESI format that is less expensive for attorneys to review".

TIP #90

The review costs associated with e-Discovery is responsible for 73% of all e-Discovery production costs.

TIP #91

Collecting the information that is needed pursuant to e-Discovery is responsible for almost 8% of expenditures.

TIP #92

Almost 19% of the costs associated with e-Discovery are related to processing the ESI.

TIP #93

Outside counsel makes up 70% of the total e-Discovery production costs.

TIP #94

Ask your atty what legal technology software (i.e. CaseMap, Summation, Catalyst Solution) they use in their law practice.

TIP #95

Ask your atty what litigation technology and legal review software platform do they use in their law practice.

TIP #96

"Some trial attorneys, with or without the permission of their clients, go so far as to enter into secret agreements with each other to ignore the [ESI]" -- Atty Ralph Losey

TIP #97

Do not engage in spoliation - - known as the negligent or intentional destruction or altercation of evidence; Otherwise, you risk facing severe consequences, including monetary sanctions, award of attorney fees, costs related to investigating and litigating the document destruction, default judgments, dismissal of certain claims or defenses, and adverse inferences to the jury about what the destroyed evidence would have shown.

TIP #98

If you think that "deleting" a document or email destroys it – then guess again. It only moves it from one sector to other undisclosed locations on the hard drive.

TIP #99

One useful acronym to remember related to receiving a litigation hold notice is: S.A.V.E.D. – Setting, Accessories, Valuable data and logs, Equipment, Disposables and packaging.

TIP #100

Protected Health Information, otherwise known as "PHI" may or may not provide automatic protection of documents and emails subject to a litigation hold notice-- even if placed in the subject line of the email.

TIP #101

A healthcare provider who may not have actual custody or possession of ESI documents – but, who can still exercise control and access to them-- still has a duty to preserve them or risk an adverse inference jury instruction and sanctions based upon alleged spoliation.

SUMMARY:

At the minimum, consider implementing the following tips using the references as a guide:

1. Create a Data map of your practice (Tip #84)

2. Create an ESI Document Retention Policy (Tip # 78)

3. Create a standardized ESI Litigation Hold Protocol (Tip #79)

4. Create an e-Discovery Checklist (Tip #80)

5. Obtain a copy of the local court rules on eDiscovery related to your specific jurisdiction / State.

References and Bibliography

Federal Government Agencies

- Centers for Medicare & Medicaid Services
- Office of Inspector General for Health & Human Services
- Code of Federal Regulations
- Department of Health & Human Services
- Federal Trade Commission
- Department of Labor

Trade Associations

- American Bar Association
- American Bar Association Health Law Section
- American College of Healthcare Executives
- American Health Information Management Association
- American Hospital Association
- American Medical Association
- American Health Lawyers Association
- American Medical Group Association
- American Society for Healthcare Risk Management
- Federation of American Hospitals
- Healthcare Finance Management Association
- Health Care Compliance Association
- Medical Group Management Association
- The Joint Commission

Websites:

http://libraryguides.missouri.edu/c.php?g=28053&p=172983

http://www.americanbar.org/publications/law_practice_home/law_practice_archive/lpm_magazine_articles_v35_is2_pg50.html

http://apps.americanbar.org/lpm/lpt/articles/slc10061.shtml

http://www.csha.info/links

Articles:

http://cornelllawreview.org/files/2013/02/Metadata-Production.pdf

http://hstlj.org/wp-content/uploads/2014/01/STLJ-Masor-Electronic-Medical-Records-and-E-Discovery.pdf

http://www.martindale.com/medical-malpractice-law/article__1517440.htm

http://www.americanbar.org/publications/law_practice_home/law_practice_archive/lpm_magazine_articles_v35_is2_pg50.html

http://www.amednews.com/article/20120917/profession/309179951/5/

http://www.law.harvard.edu/programs/plp/pdf/008-03358_03358-ch0007.pdf

http://www.babc.com/sitesearch/xpqSiteSearch.aspx?xpST=Search&qu=ediscovery&page=2

http://www.natlawreview.com/print/article/lessons-cautionary-tale-electronic-discovery-pitfalls-health-care-litigation

http://www.marshalldennehey.com/media/pdf-articles/E%20Discovery.pdf

http://www.wcl.american.edu/trial/documents/TaxationofCostsandOfferofJudgment.pdf

http://www.rand.org/pubs/monographs/MG1208.html

http://e-discoveryteam.com/school/plato%E2%80%99s-cave-why-most-lawyers-love-paper-and-hate-e-discovery-and-what-this-means-to-the-future-of-legal-education/

http://e-discoveryteam.com/2011/01/09/the-law-firm-apprenticeship-tradition-and-why-most-lawyers-are-still-untrained-in-e-discovery/

http://www.ediscoveryreadingroom.com/?p=914

http://www.lifespan.org/uploadedFiles/Lifespan/Content/Services/Winter_Insights_2013_WebEdition.pdf

http://www.gibbonslaw.com/news_publications/articles.php?action=display_publication&publication_id=2504

http://electronicdiscovery.info/e-discovery-spoliation-and-sanctions/

ELECTRONIC DISCOVERY FOR HEALTHCARE PROVIDERS written by J.S. "Chris" Christie, Jr. (Bradley Arant Rose & White LLP, Birmingham AL)

Podcasts / Video:

http://electronicdiscovery.info/e-discovery-made-simple-electronic-discovery-101/

http://electronicdiscovery.info/e-discovery-101-what-is-electronic-discovery/

https://www.youtube.com/watch?v=PqapYncB8vQ

https://www.youtube.com/watch?v=h1OZqWxEiMQ#t=13

http://esibytes.com/taxation-of-electronic-discovery-costs-recovering-processing-fees/

Medical Malpractice Litigation: The Medical and Legal Perspectives (58 min)

Books:

Saunders Medical Office Management written by Alice Anne Andress (Elsevier Health Sciences, 2013)

Source: http://www.ediscoverylaw.com/local-rules-forms-and-guidelines-of-united-states-district-courts-addressing-e-discovery-issues/ (last visited on 16 SEP 2014)

Local Rules, Forms and Guidelines of United States District Courts Addressing E-Discovery Issues

Many United States District Courts now require compliance with special local rules, forms or guidelines addressing the discovery of electronically stored information. Below is a collection of those local rules, forms and guidelines, with links to the relevant materials. Please note also that many individual judges and magistrate judges have created their own forms or have crafted their own preferred protocols for e-discovery. These are generally available on the website of the individual judge or magistrate judge and care should be taken to ensure you are aware of any such forms or guidelines in any court you may appear in.

District of Alaska
Local Rules (Civil)
Local Form 26(f): Scheduling and Planning Conference Report
Local Rule 16.1 Pre-Trial Procedures (requiring use of Local Form 26(f) or one substantially similar)

Eastern and Western Districts of Arkansas
Local Rule 26.1 Outline for Fed. R. Civ. P. 26(f) Report

Northern District of California
Guidelines for the Discovery of Electronically Stored Information
ESI Checklist for use during the Rule 26(f) meet and confer process
Model Stipulated Order Re: the Discovery of Electronically Stored Information
Standing Order for All Judges of the Northern District of California

Joint Case Management Statement & [Proposed] Order (Updated May 2013)

Guidelines for Electronic Discovery in Criminal Cases
   Electronic Discovery Protocol ("Recommendations for ESI Discovery Production in Federal Criminal Cases")
   Electronic Discovery Suggested Practices ("Suggested Practices Regarding Discovery in Complex Cases")
   Recommended E-Discovery Practices ("Recommended E-Discovery Practices for Federal Criminal Justice Act Cases")
   Initial Discovery and 3rd Party Assessment Checklist

Southern District of California
Local Rules (Scroll down to Local Patent Rules)
2.1 Governing Procedure
2.6 Model Order for Electronically Stored Information ("ESI")

Model Order Governing Discovery of Electronically Stored Information in Patent Cases

District of Colorado
Civil Case Scheduling Order

District of Connecticut
Local Rules 16(b), 26, 37 and Form 26(F)

District of Delaware
Default Standard for Discovery, Including Discovery of Electronically Stored Information ("ESI")
Default Standard for Access to Source Code

United States Bankruptcy Court, District of Delaware
Del. Bankr. L.R. 7026-3 Discovery of Electronic Documents "(E-Discovery)"

Middle District of Florida
Civil Discovery Practice Handbook (*see* Part VII "Technology")

Southern District of Florida
United States District Court for the S.D. Florida, Local Rules
Rule 16.1 Pretrial Procedure in Civil Actions
Rule 26.1 Discovery and Discovery Material (Civil)
Appendix A: Discovery Practices Handbook

Northern District of Georgia
LR 16.2 Joint Preliminary Report and Discovery Plan

Appendix B: Documents Associated with Civil Cases Pending in the United States District Court Northern District of Georgia

Southern District of Georgia
Rule 26(f) Report

United States Bankruptcy Court, District of Hawaii
LBR 1004-1. Rule 2004 Examinations

D. Idaho
Rule 16.1 Scheduling Conference, Voluntary Case Management Conference (VCM) and Litigation Plans (Choose "District (01/09/13")
(Effective Jan. 9, 2013)

Northern District of Illinois
Local Patent Rules for Electronically Stored Information

Northern District of Indiana
Report of Parties' Planning Meeting

Southern District of Indiana
Rule 16.1 Pretrial Procedures (requiring use of Uniform Case Management Plan)

Case Management Plans
Uniform Case Management Plan for Civil Cases
ESI Supplement to Report of the Parties' Planning Meeting

Uniform Patent Case Management Plans (Patents)
Phase I (Pre-Markman Ruling)
ESI Supplement to Report of the Parties Planning Meeting

Phase II (Post-Markman Ruling)

Track 3 Patent Management Plan
ESI Supplement to Report of the Parties' Planning Meeting

Northern and Southern Districts of Iowa
Scheduling Order and Discovery Plan
Instructions and Worksheet for Preparation of Scheduling Order and Discovery Plan and Order Requiring Submission of Same
Local Rule 16.1 Scheduling Order and Discovery Plan (requiring use of form)
Local Rule 26.1 Pretrial Discovery and Disclosures (requirement to submit discovery plan satisfied by submission of form Scheduling Order and Discovery Plan)

District of Kansas
Guidelines for Discovery of Electronically Stored Information

Initial Order Regarding Planning and Scheduling (scroll to Civil Forms)

District of Maryland
Suggested Protocol for Discovery of Electronically Stored Information

Local Rules
Rule 802 Scheduling Conference
Stipulated Order Regarding Confidentiality of Discovery Material and Inadvertent Disclosure of Privileged Material
Appendix A: Discovery Guidelines of the United States District Court for the District of Maryland

United States Bankruptcy Court, District of Maryland
Appendix C: Discovery Guidelines of the United States District for the District of Maryland

District of Massachusetts
Local Rule 16.6 Scheduling and Procedures in Patent Infringement Cases

District of Minnesota
Local Rules of Civil Procedure
Form 3 Rule 26(f) Report
Form 4 Rule 26(f) Report (Patent Cases)

Northern and Southern Districts of Mississippi
Local Uniform Civil Rules
Rule 26 Discovery Control
Rule 45 Subpoena
Case Management Order

Eastern District of Missouri
Rule 26-3.01 Federal Rule of Civil Procedure 26

District of Nebraska
Form 35: Report of Parties' Rule 26(f) Planning Conference

District of New Hampshire
Local Rule 26.1 Discovery Plan
Civil Form 2: Sample Discovery Plan

District of New Jersey
Local Rule 26.1 Discovery (*see* subpart (d))

Joint Proposed Discovery Plan

Eastern District of New York
Local Rule 26.3 Uniform Definitions in Discovery Requests

Northern District of New York
General Order 25 (see subsection G of Case Management Plan form)

Southern District of New York
Local Rule 26.3 Uniform Definitions in Discovery Requests

Standing Order (In re: Pilot Project Regarding Case Management Techniques for Complex Civil Cases in the Southern District of New York [*see in particular*, Exhibit B: Joint Electronic Submission and Proposed Order])

Western District of New York
Rule 16 Alternative Dispute Resolution and Pretrial Conferences
Rule 26 General Rules Governing Discovery

Local Patent Rules
Rule 2. General Provisions
[Model] Order Regarding e-Discovery in Patent Cases

Western District of North Carolina
Local Civil Rule 16.1 Pretrial Conferences (see subpart (G) Initial Pretrial Conference)

Northern District of Ohio
Local Rules, Appendix K: Default Standards for Discovery of Electronically Stored Information ("E-Discovery")

Rule 16.3 Track Assignment and Case Management Conference

Local Patent Rules
Appendix A: Stipulated Protective Order
Appendix B: Report of Parties' Planning Meeting in Patent Cases

Southern District of Ohio
Rule 26(f) Report of Parties (Western Division at Dayton)
Rule 26(f) Report of the Parties (Eastern Division)

General Order No. 12-01. Pretrial and Trial Procedures [Dayton]

Northern District of Oklahoma
Guidelines for Discovery of Electronically Stored Information

Western District of Oklahoma
Appendix II, Form: Joint Status Report and Discovery Plan (Choose "Civil and Criminal, scroll to relevant Appendix [p. 71])

LCrR 16.1 Discovery Conference
Best Practices for Electronic Discovery of Documentary Materials in Criminal Cases

District of Oregon
LR 26-6 E-Discovery in Patent Cases
Model Order Regarding E-Discovery in Patent Cases

Eastern District of Pennsylvania
Report of Rule 26(f) Meeting

Middle District of Pennsylvania
26.1 Duty to Investigate and Disclose
Appendix A Joint Case Management Plan

Western District of Pennsylvania
Local Rules of Court (See Local Civil Rules)
Local Rule 16.1 Pretrial Procedures
Local Rule 26.2 Discovery of Electronically Stored Information
Local Rule 34 Serving and Responding to Requests for Production in Electronic Form

Appendix 16.1A: 26(f) Report of the Parties
Appendix 23.E: 26(f) Joint Report of the Parties (Class Action)

U.S. Bankruptcy Court for the Western District of Pennsylvania
Local Rules of the U.S. Bankruptcy Court for the Western District of Pennsylvania
7026-1 Discovery of Electronic Documents ("E-Discovery")
7026-2 Electronic Discovery Special Master

District of Puerto Rico
Rule 16 Pretrial Conferences; Scheduling; Management

Middle District of Tennessee
Administrative Order No. 174: Default Standard for Discovery of Electronically Stored
Information ("E-Discovery")

Western District of Tennessee
Local Rules: Civil
Local Rule 26.1 Discovery in Civil Cases
Appendix G LR 16.2 Track 3 (Expedited) Scheduling Order
Appendix H LR 16.2 Track 4 (Standard) Scheduling Order
Appendix I LR 16.2 Track 5 (Complex) Scheduling Order

Local Patent Rules
Appendix A: Stipulated Patent Case Protective Order
Appendix B: Joint Planning Report and Proposed Schedule

Eastern District of Texas
[Model] Order Regarding E-Discovery in Patent Cases (see Appendix P)

Northern District of Texas
Amended Miscellaneous Order No. 62 (Dallas Division, Patent Cases) (*see* item 2.1(a)(2))

Southern District of Texas
Local Rules of Practice for Patent Cases Rule 2-1. Procedure

District of Utah
Attorney's Planning Meeting Report

United States Bankruptcy Court, District of Utah
Form 35: Report of the Parties' Planning Meeting Pursuant to Fed. R. Civ. P. 26(f)

District of Vermont
Rule 26. Discovery

Western District of Washington
Local Rules of Civil Procedure

Rule 26 Duty to Disclose; General Provisions Governing Discovery
(Effective Dec. 1, 2012)
Model Agreement Regarding Discovery of Electronically Stored Information (as addressed in LR 26(f)(1)(I)(ii).
(Effective Dec. 1, 2012)

CrR 16. Discovery and Inspection

Southern District of West Virginia
Report of Parties' Planning Meeting
Local Rule 16.1 Scheduling Conferences (requiring use of court's form)

Eastern District of Wisconsin
Civil L. R. 16 Pretrial Conferences; Scheduling; Management; Alternative Dispute Resolution
Civil L. R. 26 Duty to Disclose; General Provisions Governing Discovery

District of Wyoming
Local Civil Rules
26.1 Discovery
26.2 Electronically Stored Information (ESI)

United States Court of Appeals Seventh Circuit
Electronic Discovery Pilot Program

Other:
Recommendations for Electronically Stored Information (ESI) Discovery Production in Federal Criminal Cases (developed by the Department of Justice/Administrative Office Joint Working Group of Electronic Technology JETWG])

For more information on the local rules of United States District Courts, click here to see a page with links to all the District Courts' web pages.